NOURISHING NUTRITION™

Reclaim your health and vitality.

Reap the bountiful rewards while eating as nature intended.
Claim your health and vitality with these simple,
yet powerful tools to nourish and heal your body.

NOURISHING NUTRITION COPYRIGHT

Please note:

The written or spoken information, ideas, procedures and suggestions contained and presented in 'NOURISHING NUTRITION' workshops and books are meant for educational purposes only and are not for diagnosis. It should not be used as a substitute for your physician's advice. 'NOURISHING NUTRITION' is not therapy and is not intended to replace the recommendations of a licensed health practitioner. It is the responsibility of the reader to consult with their own medical Doctor, Counselor, Therapist or other competent professional regarding any condition before adopting any of the suggestions in this book.

NOURISHING NUTRITION™

*Dedicated to the innate wisdom of the body,
which is endlessly devoted to our health,
vitality and life force.*

MISSION STATEMENT

To guide and facilitate women
in becoming their most beautiful and radiant selves.

To acknowledge and embrace the well of love
and power which lies within all women and to ignite the
awakening and embodying of this life force.

To empower each woman, through exquisite self-care and love,
to live her fullest life possible, and to walk her path of wisdom
and truth, as she shares this light and knowledge
with all beings.

IN DEEP GRATITUDE

thank you

The creation, birth and life of 'A Woman's Truth' would not have been possible without the love, support and devotion from the following angels in my life:

My beautiful daughter Megan who naturally embodies the teachings of living in her truth and integrity, thank you for the creative gift of the beautiful artwork. Helena Nelson-Reed for her generosity of spirit in allowing her extraordinary artwork, which embodies the teachings so magnificently, to grace the covers. Dennise Marie Keller for her unwavering support and dedication to the teachings and for proofing, editing, aligning and translating my vision into the technical world of manifestation. Dan Fowler for his creative genius and dedication. Lucy Alexander and Suzanne Ryan, my dearest friends for their amazing editing and wholehearted encouragement. Monica Marsh for her commitment, support and belief in the workshops. Maggie Crawford, my mum, for her proofing and for being a living example of the teachings. Cait Myer and Katie Steen for their patience and ability to decipher my handwriting and for formatting the books. Bethany Kelly for her support. Deborah Waring for holding the space for the conception of 'A Woman's Truth' to be born and for her insight in the first year of teaching and Emmanuel for believing in my vision.

My mentors and teachers Rod Stryker, Adyashanti and Alison Armstrong, Max Simon and Jeffrey Van Dyk for their continuous and guiding light in my life, their never-ending belief in my potential and for always teaching me the way to evolve into my highest and most potent self. And to all of you beautiful and courageous women who are committing to living your truth and transforming into your most radiant selves,

thank you.

A PRELUDE

An overture to Nourishing Nutrition.

Eating is one of the highest pleasures of being human, and can be a source of strength and nourishment, or a tormented experience for those who struggle with food and the compulsions surrounding it.

Eating is a choice that we make more often than many other choices in life. We have three to five opportunities to choose well every day, that is 35 choices a week or 1,050 choices in a month.

Entering into a state of mindfulness with food, from what goes into the grocery cart to what we chop and prepare, to chewing and assimilation, can create a relationship with food that is nourishing, grounding and healing.

The art of cooking has been displaced by the ease of eating out and convenience foods as working women do their best to keep pace with multiple competing priorities. It is difficult to maintain health and truly know what is in your food when others are preparing it for you. It is the act of cooking that is empowering and eating simple, whole foods is the road back to alignment with our food, an our bodies.

In the busy milieu of today's society, many women have lost touch with their sense of what it is to be strong and healthy in their bodies. We tend to focus on only a small aspect of nutrition, or a certain supplement, gleaning health information from the internet, friends, attempting radical cleanses followed by a return to more processed foods before we know it. Good intentions are thrown in with the pace of modern life, family and career, hoping it works.

The truth is, it is not one aspect of diet that leads to health, and there are no magic foods that effortlessly release weight from your body. I wish that is was that simple!

The keys to vibrant health and a beautiful relationship with food are to tap into what foods nourish *you,* what amounts of those foods are best for *you* and then once and for all, declare a truce on the war with food and your body.

Miranda Barrett's book '*Nourishing Nutrition*' is an inspiring work that encourages women to build up their stores of self-love, releasing the use of will power to heal their relationship with food. She uses transparent story telling that relays the wisdom she has learned in her own relationship with food, coupled with factual wisdom on nutrition and health.

To read '*Nourishing Nutrition*' feels as if you are sitting at the kitchen table with the author, being fed a soup to soothe your soul, an entrée to build your spirit and a dessert to release you from guilt and old patterns.

'*Nourishing Nutrition*' is a compendium of knowledge, inspiration and truth that serves as a much needed guide for all seeking to recalibrate their relationship to food and reclaim their vitality as healthy, balanced women.

~ Nicole Fox, MPH, RDN
Registered Dietitian Nutritionist & Integrative Health Coach

NOURISHING NUTRITION™

Gems of Truth

You can download a copy of **An Honest Daily Food Study**

from Miranda's website at

www.MirandaJBarrett.com/ resources/nourishing-nutrition

A DAILY PRACTICE

commit to Yourself

*F*ollow these simple steps daily as a way to instill and strengthen your heartfelt resolve to love yourself. This will help to keep you aligned, transforming and on track, giving you a stable foundation for the rest of your life. As a gift to yourself, please mark the teachings as you read them through and congratulate yourself with each one. See each day as a commitment to take exquisite care of yourself.

You can download a copy of **An Honest Daily Food Study**

from Miranda's website at

www.MirandaJBarrett.com/ resources/nourishing-nutrition

A LIFE WORTH LIVING

"Never give from your well.
Always give from your overflow."
~Rumi

All too often as women, your own needs are denied for the benefit of others as you orchestrate your life through demands and expectations you feel responsible for. Unfortunately, this can leave you without the juice and energy needed to be present fully and to enjoy life. During these readings, you will continually discover more about who you truly are and learn the tools needed to live your most authentic and fulfilling life possible. From this place, you will experience being 'full to overflowing' and all the joy and energy this brings.

As you delve into these teachings, you will explore, laugh, study, share, and freely express who you are. In this sacred space, you will ultimately learn your truth as a woman in order to shine, to embody your own beauty, believe in your own worth, and take exquisite care of yourself. For only in this way can you truly be of service.

During these guidebooks, many of the basic needs of women will be explored such as sleep, nutrition, creativity, movement and time to replenish. A topic has been chosen for each book and a cohesive and practical foundation is laid out to inspire and guide you. This will bring about a new strength and resolve which will allow your needs to become a priority, without letting your outer world dictate otherwise. By the end of our time together, the concept of being confident, loving, serene and passionate will no longer be a distant fantasy. Instead, these and many other extraordinary qualities that you naturally embody as a woman will flow with ease, grace and love.

With life's demands so high, it has become imperative that your needs are first acknowledged, honored and then taken care of. From this vantage point, your relationship with yourself then has the potential to be transformed into one of self-love. The beauty is this in turn creates a life that not only fulfills you and your life's purpose, but also allows everyone touched by your presence to receive this gift.

I look forward to spending this precious time with you.

Welcome to A Woman's Truth.

Sincerely and with love,

Miranda

NOURISHING NUTRITION

We are what we eat.

*T*here are many reasons for human beings to eat. Some of the motivations are extremely practical, such as you die without food and it provides the body with essential fuel. Other reasons can be deeply emotional, like the need to comfort yourself with eating. On the other hand, perhaps, you consume food or drink because you seek stimulation or escape. The good news is that once you become aware of some of your personal triggers, you can consciously choose to handle them more appropriately. Unfortunately, if you allow yourself to eat without thinking, you may gravitate towards food, which is unhealthy.

FOOD FOR SURVIVAL

The body's fuel.

Food and water are one of the four basic human survival needs. Everyone has to eat and drink in order to live. Without physical nourishment the body dies. Therefore, the human DNA is programmed to need desire and search for food.

The reason for this programming is that the cells in the body need nourishment. Obviously, it is hard for a tiny blood cell to receive iron from a bowl of spinach that is sitting on a plate. Consequently, the body is designed to break down the food into tiny particles, allowing each and every cell to receive exactly what it needs. The old adage 'we are what we eat' is accurate. Whatever you ingest is transported to your cells, which make up your body and provide your health and your energy.

The design of the human body is quite miraculous. Both food and sex have the possibility of being extremely pleasurable. There is a reason for this. Because pleasure is derived from both of these desires, it is natural to seek them out, thus keeping the body alive and the species reproducing. Never underestimate the power of your survival instinct. It is often the driving force behind much of what you do on a daily basis.

Another interesting part of this survival-based need is how much time, energy and money is spent on food and drink. Just notice as you drive around, how many buildings are designated for the production, consumption or marketing of food. It is hard not to notice the dominance of food in this culture. Much time is spent planning the next meal and the next taste-experience. This has become an integral part of life today.

"Each year when spring comes I choose to cleanse. Just as spring-cleaning is in the air, my body becomes part of this ritual. One of the cleanses I choose involves a drink of lemon juice, cayenne pepper, maple syrup and water—that is it. For a number of days, this is all that I ingest. After the third day, a strange phenomenon begins: I start to feel good. I have battled through the detoxification part and now I feel clear, pleasantly empty, calm and strangely energized. One of the biggest gifts is that I no longer have to think about food. For a time, I do not have to shop, plan, cook or clean up. All that energy can be spent elsewhere. Obviously I eventually need to start eating again, but the pause in the momentum of eating is often a wonderful vacation." ~ Miranda

FOOD AND EMOTIONS

what we eat affects how we feel,
and how we feel affects what we eat.

When you eat junk food, which is basically devoid of all life-force and vitality, you are essentially choosing to disconnect from life. By ingesting dead food, you are literally robbing yourself of the goodness, energy and joy that real, live and vibrant foods can provide. Unfortunately, the choice to eat processed foods not only causes a distorted reaction in the body, but also allows you to carry on as the living-dead. Just think about it: how different do you feel when you eat a big bountiful salad for lunch versus some French fries or a candy bar? Which one sustains you and gives you life force? Which one has vitality still growing in it? Which one nourishes you?

For some people, eating dead food can actually facilitate and keep their depression and misery alive. It can support a negative reality and keep it going. Food really can be the perfect medicine. By eating live, nutritious foods, you will feel more vibrant and outgoing. The choice to eat well will actually bring you out of survival mode, giving the message to the body that there are choices and plenty of food to go around. This brings you back to a sense of abundance, gratitude and a feeling that your life is in harmony with nature.

"Over the years I have met people who seem to have no emotional connection to food. They eat when they are hungry and stop when they are satisfied. Well this was certainly not my path. I love food. I love its taste, its smell and the feeling of a full belly. I have also noticed that my emotions play a part in how I eat. Even though I long for the simplicity of being an unemotional eater, in reality this is not my path. I have to be supremely conscious about choosing to eat out of my physical need for food, rather than using it as a reward or a source of stimulation or avoidance."
~ Miranda

FOOD AS AN ESCAPE

Choosing not to feel.

Eating or over eating is one of the most powerful and effective tools available to suppress emotions. Obviously, there are times when a pain or upset is so intense, that you actually feel nauseous and lose your appetite or have no desire to eat at all.

Sometimes, however, you might use food as an anesthetic, to numb a chronic problem. You may then compound this situation by listening to your internal critic, who beats you up for eating the fourth cookie. The result is a suppressed emotion, a sugar high and a dose of self-loathing - not a pretty picture.

Another and more courageous choice is to feel the emotion that got the ball rolling in the first place. Knowing that, as with all feelings, it will eventually pass.

FOOD AS A REWARD

I deserve another cookie!

How often have you walked to the fridge or cupboard looking for a treat? You are not hungry, yet you feel you deserve something special after working all day and giving your all. Unfortunately, a tub of ice cream then becomes that something special and represents the recognition you seek, the 'you-time' you crave. However, this is a sure sign that you are trading food for actually giving yourself credit for what you have accomplished that day.

If food has become the reward, be open to choosing a different prize. Maybe a hot bath, a foot rub or a night on the town could do the trick. Find your own medicine and give it to yourself. Food chosen as a treat tends not to be the healthiest and is often eaten later in the day. This then leads to other problems, such as not being able to sleep and weight gain. The good news is that good sex, a satisfying book or movie is calorie free.

FOOD AS STIMULATION

Eating out of boredom.

Another classic reason for emotional eating is boredom. You need some excitement. Maybe it has been a rather mundane day and one of the quickest and easiest fixes is to stimulate your taste buds. Note the word stimulation here. What this means is that steamed broccoli will not cut it, but fried, salty, crispy or sweet food will. Again, you are back in the danger zone of unhealthy choices.

Have you ever noticed when you are engrossed in something, you forget to eat, drink and even pee? This is because in those moments your passion and desire override your survival instinct for nourishment. Therefore, if you are finding that, at certain times of the day, you are gravitating towards food, even though you are not hungry, you need to inquire if there is enough creativity and passion in your life. Take the beginning of a sexual relationship for instance, when your appetite disappears. Suddenly sex is much more appealing than cake. There is a clue here!

FOOD AS PROTECTION

Gaining weight can be a very powerful way to insulate and protect.

The compulsion to overeat can be an effective way to add an extra layer of protection. The trigger in this situation is survival-based. If the brain, psyche or body feels unsafe and is threatened by the possibility of famine or starvation, it has its own innate intelligence to gather extra fat cells in case they might be needed later. This is one of the reasons that while pregnant, a woman will gain some extra body weight, therefore she and the baby will be able to survive longer in a disaster situation.

It is also interesting to note that during times of economic crisis, some people will react to the stress of this situation by gaining weight. It will not be a conscious decision, yet the gradual build-up of pounds will be evident. Unfortunately, this brilliant survival mechanism goes awry when overeating is activated out of emotional fear. This trigger is not about physical starvation, but a belief that your emotional well-being is being threatened. In this scenario, there is possibly a belief that a certain situation or person is not safe and the only way to protect yourself is to have a physical buffer between you. I am referring to physical body fat. For some women, weight gain can also result in a feeling of being isolated and shut down. In a way, it can give you permission to not show up and live life fully. This needing protection dance moves beautifully to the music of food as a reward, an escape or stimulation, which is a lethal combination.

"There have been times in my life when I have not wanted to be in a relationship or to have to deal with unwanted attention from men. It has usually been when some old wound is raising its ugly head and I am not willing to move through it yet. Over the years, I have chosen different modalities to isolate myself. They have ranged from shaving my head, wearing asexual clothes, not smiling, to gaining a chunk of weight. I used to treat myself like my worst enemy. You know that voice in the head. Nowadays I choose to love myself whatever my weight. It has been a challenge and is a continuous conscious decision. Yet, the triggers to gaining the weight are still present. The difference is I no longer judge and berate myself. The journey I walk with the extra poundage becomes a sweeter and gentler one filled with love and compassion, rather than self-loathing and disgust." ~ Miranda

WILL FUELLED BY LOVE FOR THE SELF

Practice is the path.

In an ideal world, eating healthy nutritious food would not only be desirable, but effortless. Eating only when hungry would be completely natural and saying no to the sugary delicious dessert would be obvious.

In our dreams...

What is it that needs to be cultivated when your world is not so perfect? When you are tired, rushed, stressed, hungry or depressed, stimulating or fast food will seem like the only option. The question is what else you could rely on in order to get through that moment, so another choice can be made.

One possible answer is '**will-power**'.

The following are some definitions of the word '**will**':

◆   The power to choose what you will do.

◆   The combination of determination and self-discipline
     that enables somebody to do something despite the difficulties involved.

Will power is the drive that gets you up in the morning to go to work even when you do not feel like it. Will power is what is needed to take actions when you do not necessarily want to. Therefore, a good question to ask at this point would be:

How do you cultivate a strong will?

There may well have been times in your life when you have felt highly motivated. For a while not eating sugar and exercising regularly felt attainable and rewarding. Yet, have you noticed how, over time, this momentum sometimes wanes and you slip back into your old habits? What is it that would keep this will alive?

It seems as though the motivating factor behind will power is often the force needed to feed and energize it. Self-love is one of the most powerful motivating factors.

When it comes to nutrition, it is a completely different scenario to eat well because you think you are overweight and unattractive. The alternative is to make healthy choices because you will then feel good, have more energy and feel happier and calmer. A loving approach will fuel your motivation for many miles and days to come, while self-loathing will probably mean that you soon lose heart and give up trying to eat healthily. Given the choice between a supportive and loving advocate or a mean and critical bitch, which one would you want by your side?

The trouble begins when self-love and self-loathing are at odds and it is not clear which is the motivating factor. A simple way to fathom which is which is to ask:

Is this a loving act towards myself?

This will be obvious if the action needed will provide a benefit for you. Where it can be confusing is when you are choosing to be of service to others. Unless your well is full to overflowing and you have the energy, resources and time to be of service to that person or situation, it is not an act of love. Unfortunately, when you are forcing yourself to be there for others, the result is often depletion, resentment, anger and exhaustion. Obviously, the momentum behind the will that pushed you through was not loving to your needs and could possibly be harmful to yourself.

Therefore, before you embark on any great changes in your life, be mindful to look at your motivating factor first.

Ask Yourself:

why do I want to make this transformation?

If the inspiration is positive, such as you want to feel better, then chances are you will be able to sustain the new vision. This love for yourself will fuel the **will** that is needed to keep you on track, because the force behind it is loving and promotes your well-being.

Spend some time creating a loving approach to any change that you are making. In this context, the topic is about food, yet this philosophy can be extended to exercise, getting enough sleep and having some downtime.

"In my experience, if I do not exercise regularly, I become tired and tend to crave sugar. Because I have less energy my body then goes on a rampage searching for a quick fix and sugar or caffeine are obvious, yet detrimental, solutions. A more loving approach would be to go to bed earlier!" ~ Miranda

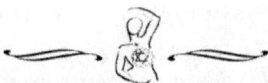

"When a human soul draws its first furrow straight, the rest will surely follow."
~ Anonymous

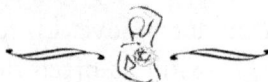

MARRIAGE OF RHYTHM AND WILL

Following life's rhythm.

When you are out of rhythm with your truth, it is frequently your will which keeps you going, often to the point of exhaustion. Yet when you are in balance with your own truth and authenticity, there is a tendency to fall into a natural rhythm. Life then becomes less of an effort and your will can be used as an advocate to support your desires, rather than forcing you through your denials.

Life is rather like a dance, often being led by conditioned responses. Sometimes these reactions can dominate and set your wants and needs aside for the benefit of others. This imbalance gives your will the responsibility to carry you through these programmed beliefs, yet at the same time unfortunately depleting your mind, body and soul. Your energy is then used to sustain the will power it takes to accomplish these actions, which may not necessarily support your natural rhythm or truth.

When utilized for your highest good, will power does not leave you drained. In contrast, it supports your ability to live in your truth.

◆ How often is your will in direct opposition to the natural rhythm of your life?

◆ When does your will have to take over because you are exhausted?

◆ How often are you denying what feels right within the rhythm of life?

Your physical body requires nutrition, and so does your emotional body. Eating stimulating or numbing foods deeply influences your emotional state and vice versa. When emotions are running wild it can strongly influence your food choices.

"I am always amazed to witness my gravitational pull to comforting, and usually not so healthy foods when I am emotional. The days before my period, all I want are sweets and chocolate. When I am feeling hurt, I crave cheese! Feeling overwhelmed seems to stimulate a strong desire for fatty foods. I am sure there is some great logic to all of this. Sweet foods expand the body and help the womb to open up. Chocolate contains magnesium, and fats feed the brain and give energy. Yet all I know is that I feel like a crazy woman on a food rampage." ~ Miranda

This is a journey of discovery as you learn to discern your own personal triggers and comfort foods and learn about their impact on you. As you become more aware of how your body feels, you will notice when you begin to grow lethargic or your stomach is upset. You may even feel depressed or agitated because of what you have eaten. Instead of ignoring these symptoms, listen to the messages. They are your body's way of saying it is out of alignment with the truth of what you need.

Good nutrition always begins with a conscious choice.

Nature has her own beautiful and natural rhythm when it comes to food and when your will is aligned with this natural intelligence, you receive all the vitality you need. Honor yourself, speak your truth, and nourish all of who you are: your body, your mind and your spirit.

Choose to pledge allegiance to your own rhythm, will and deeper truths.

THE FOOD OF LIFE

Better health.

*E*veryone eats, perhaps three or four times a day and food is placed in your mouth for a variety of reasons. So, just how important is the food you eat? Hopefully, hunger is the main one, yet sometimes, boredom or comfort may come in as a close second. Food is your body's fuel. Like any well-oiled machine, the body needs energy from food, water and air in order to survive and survive it will on very little.

The human body is an amazing instrument.

It will tolerate great abuse, continual consumption of junk and processed food, polluted air or water, inadequate rest and large quantities of drugs, stimulants and stress. But at some point the overload light will go on and the body will no longer be able to function the way it did. Illness will set in and if there is no change in lifestyle, these destructive habits may lead to death. This is not about cheating death, but about improving the quality of your life.

What does a change in lifestyle mean? Do you need more money? Do you need to leave your job? Do you need to spend less time studying? No! The changes required are subtle. You already eat and drink. The transitions could be as small as having a bottle of water instead of a soda, using a pinch of sea salt instead of regular salt or eating an apple instead of a candy bar. Mainly, it is about taking control of your body and what you put into it. Through advertising and social pressures, you may have lost faith in your own choices. The power has been given over to the media, to doctors and to convenience. You no longer listen to your own inner voice, which would naturally choose a plate of vegetables instead French fries.

By eating a diet rich in vegetables and whole grains, low in saturated fats and processed food, high in good quality oil, protein and fruits, your body will thrive. It will work at its optimum levels because it is receiving what it needs. You will have more energy and clarity of mind. You will no longer be on the continual roller coaster ride of sugar and caffeine-fuelled highs and lows. By eliminating refined and processed foods and eating organic produce in its natural state, your body will no longer have to work to overcome its intake of toxins.

Instead, that energy can go towards life.
Be gentle with yourself on this journey towards better health.

Make any changes gradually, maybe one or two at a time. When the transformation feels comfortable, move along. Be kind and do not beat yourself up for the odd sugar fix. Use the experience to notice how it makes you feel and know each step you take is in the right direction. Every journey begins with a single step.

This is your gift waiting to happen...

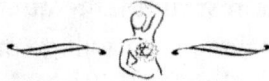

"The food you choose
can either be a medicine
or a poison. Choose wisely."
~ Anonymous

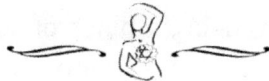

NUTRITION INQUIRY

By bringing consciousness to unconscious acts,
new habits can be formed and health and vitality restored.

Becoming aware of the choices you make around food can have a huge impact on your emotions, your energy levels and your overall sense of well-being. You may have already noticed how difficult it is to remain calm, patient and loving when you are starving or wired on a caffeine or a sugar high. The old adage 'we are what we eat' can also be translated into 'our reactions are a result of what we eat'.

◆ Do you eat?

   ◊ Breakfast?

   ◊ Lunch?

   ◊ Dinner?

◆ Do you skip meals?

   ◊ Yes   ◊ No

◆ Do you get cranky when you are hungry?

   ◊ Yes   ◊ No

◆ Do your energy levels drop when you are hungry?

   ◊ Yes   ◊ No

◆ Do you sit down to eat? (The car and your desk do not count!)

   ◊ Yes   ◊ No

◈ **Do you multi-task while eating?**
Such as driving, watching television, standing at the kitchen counter or talking on the phone.

◊ Yes ◊ No

◈ **Do you drink water?**

◊ Yes ◊ No

◈ **How many glasses a day?**

◈ **Do you drink liquids with your meals?**

◊ Yes ◊ No

◈ **Do you drink iced drinks with meals?**

◊ Yes ◊ No

◈ **What is your first drink of the day?**

◈ **What is your largest meal of the day?**

◊ Breakfast?

◊ Lunch?

◊ Dinner?

◆ What is your medium-sized meal of the day?

    ◊ Breakfast?

    ◊ Lunch?

    ◊ Dinner?

◆ What is your smallest meal of the day?

    ◊ Breakfast?

    ◊ Lunch?

    ◊ Dinner?

◆ Do you diet?

    ◊ Yes   ◊ No

◆ Has dieting had the long lasting effect you desired?

    ◊ Yes   ◊ No

◆ Do you consciously pay attention to what you put in your mouth?

    ◊ Yes   ◊ No

◆ Do you snack, nibble or graze?

    ◊ Yes   ◊ No

◆ Are you conscious of how much you are snacking on?

    ◊ Yes   ◊ No

◆ Do you find yourself snacking on junk food?

◊ Yes   ◊ No

◆ Do you eat vegetables?

◊ With breakfast?
◊ With lunch?
◊ With dinner?
◊ As snacks?

◆ Do you eat fruit?

◊ With breakfast?
◊ With lunch?
◊ With dinner?
◊ As snacks?

◆ Do you eat refined sugar?

◊ Yes   ◊ No

◆ How many times a day?

◆ Do you drink soda?

◊ Yes   ◊ No

◆ How many times a day?

◆ Do you drink caffeinated drinks?

◇ Yes   ◇ No

◆ How many times a day?

◆ Do you drink alcohol?

◇ Yes   ◇ No

◆ How much?

◆ Do you use artificial sweeteners?

◇ Yes   ◇ No

◆ Do you use sea salt?

◇ Yes   ◇ No

◆ Do you eat unhealthy fats such as hydrogenated oils?

◇ Yes   ◇ No

◆ Are you sensitive to perfumes, chemicals and smoke?

  ◊ Yes   ◊ No

◆ Do you bloat after eating?

  ◊ Yes   ◊ No

◆ How do you feel after eating?

  ◊ Satisfied
  ◊ Full
  ◊ Exhausted
  ◊ Energized
  ◊ Still craving something to eat
  ◊ Want something sweet

◆ Does your energy level drop around three or four in the afternoon?

  ◊ Yes   ◊ No

◆ Do you have sugar cravings, as though you are possessed?

  ◊ Yes   ◊ No

◆ Do you have a bowel movement every day?

  ◊ Yes   ◊ No

◈ What color is your urine?

◊ Clear ◊ Pale ◊ Yellow

◈ How many times do you urinate a day?

◈ Do you view your relationship with food as?

◊ A necessity

◊ A comfort

◊ A punishment

◊ An obsession

◊ A deprivation

◊ A means to an end

◊ A reward

◊ A joy

◊ A way to keep control

◊ All or nothing

◈ If you were to eliminate one of your favorite comfort food groups, how do you think you would you react?

◈ What do you feel you would need to support this transition?

ONE DAY AT A TIME

It is not what we eat occasionally
that causes problems, it is what we eat every day.

Change is best accomplished in a series of slow and gradual steps. As new healthy habits are formed, the desire to revert to old, undesirable behavior will diminish. It has been said that the first time you do something it is a choice, yet after a few repetitions it becomes a habit that you no longer question. The goal is to break away from the unconscious habits that may be harming you.

It is easiest to add new foods gradually to your existing way of eating, while slowly eliminating unhealthy comfort foods. Once the body becomes more balanced with the influx of nutrients, strong cravings for sugars and refined carbohydrates will begin to subside. Using higher quality substitutes is one of the easiest ways to start your new program. For example, buying organic, unrefined olive oil will increase the quality and nutritional value of any dish.

Nature moves in incremental steps. A flower does not just blossom. It moves from a seed to a tiny bud to an unfolding bloom. Its blossoming is a process, just as your life is a journey.

Change can feel overwhelming when you attempt to fix too much at once. Remember, life happens one step at a time.

Take heart...or possibly, assume a change of heart.

Start by adding in healthier and live foods such as plenty of fresh fruits and vegetables. If you feel satisfied with a delicious meal of high quality protein and plenty of tasty fresh vegetables, you may not even desire a dessert. This is because the body is already sated. Yet, if you are snacking your way through your day without pausing to eat and not getting enough nutrients, your body will keep craving and searching for what it needs and you all know where that can lead…

The following simple guidelines are stepping-stones to creating healthy changes in your life and eating habits.

◈ Try one and see how it feels.

◈ When you are comfortable, add another.

It is what you add versus what you avoid that will restore your health.

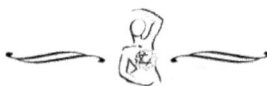

"whatever choices you make,
will either add to your health and vitality
or take away from it."
~ Anonymous

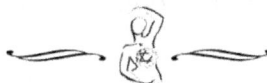

GOLDEN RULES TO EAT BY

One choice at a time.

The following are some golden rules to live by when it comes to eating consciously and well. They will help keep you on this side of the cookie jar and away from the choices, which can tend to spiral into uncontrolled eating.

◆ **Drink plenty of pure, room temperature water between meals.**

◊ No more than half a cup of liquid should be consumed during a meal; otherwise, it dilutes the digestive enzymes to break down food.

◊ Ice cold drinks slow down digestion.

◊ Be sure to hydrate the body by drinking plenty of water upon waking.

◊ The Kangan Water Machine and System is highly recommended.

◆ **Always eat a hearty breakfast.**

This is never a meal to skip. As the word suggests, it is breaking the fast and is a vital part of switching on the body's metabolism providing you with enough energy for the day ahead.

◆ **Sit down to eat in a calm, relaxed environment.**

Eating while nervous or stressed greatly inhibits the body's ability to digest food. This does not include eating in the car or in front of the refrigerator!

◆ Try to finish eating by 7 p.m.

This allows the body time to digest, burn calories and then rest until the following day. It also helps with losing weight and promotes being able to fall asleep easily and stay in a deep sleep.

◆ Avoid multi-tasking while eating.

This means you pay more attention to what you are putting into your mouth. While standing at the kitchen counter snacking, it is extraordinary how much food you can consume without even noticing it.

◆ Increase your intake of organic, fresh vegetables.

For delicious ideas, please see recipes from 'Food Of Life, The Versatile Vegetable' cookbook by Miranda Barrett.

Please go to www.MirandaJBarrett.com/resources/nourishing-nutrition

◆ Build up your supply of friendly bacteria with pro-biotic powders, pills or foods like yogurt, keifer, apple cider vinegar, kombucha, or cultured foods.

◊ These food choices will help with sugar cravings and your overall health, including your immune system, hormones, digestion and even your mood.

◊ They are especially beneficial after stressful situations such as eating rich meals, fast foods or preservatives and after taking prescription drugs, antibiotics or birth control pills.

◆ **Increase your daily intake of high quality fiber.**

    ◊ Fiber is important because it helps to relieve constipation.

    ◊ It reduces cholesterol and the desire to overeat.

    ◊ Fiber also slows down the absorption of sugar into the blood stream, leveling your energy supply.

    ◊ Freshly ground flax seed is an excellent source of fiber. It tastes good, contains healthy fats, can decrease inflammation and blood sugar levels, and has been known to help with hot flashes.

    ◊ It is recommended to start with one teaspoon of ground flax seed a day and gradually increase the amount up to a tablespoon; the digestive system can then adjust to the intake of more fiber. The flax seed can be mixed with an 8oz glass of water. Make sure you drink it immediately as it tends to solidify. It can also be sprinkled over oatmeal, yogurt, cereals, smoothies, soups, salads and is excellent in baked goods.

◆ **Eliminate refined white sugars.**

    ◊ White sugar contains no nutritional value and actually steals nutrients from the body in order to be absorbed and processed.

    ◊ If you are craving sugar, eat more protein and plenty of pro-biotics.

    ◊ Use natural sweeteners, such as Stevia, Xylitol or Lohan.

    ◊ Grade B maple syrup, agave nectar, raw honey, date sugar, palm sugar or rice syrup can also be good replacements if your digestion is strong and there is no sign of Candida or yeast infections.

◆ **Switch to a high quality sea salt.**

Celtic, Himalayan or Real salt are all excellent choices.

◆ **Reduce intake of white refined flour.**

    ◊ White refined flour is similar to refined sugar in the way that it breaks down in the body and has no nutritional value.

    ◊ Try substituting with whole grains and gluten-free products.

◆ **Read food labels and pay attention to the ingredients in drinks.**

Avoid:

    ◊ High fructose corn syrup

    ◊ Hydrogenated and partially hydrogenated oils and trans fats

    ◊ Refined, enriched and fortified products

    ◊ Processed foods

    ◊ Nitrates and nitrites

    ◊ Artificial sweeteners

    ◊ Artificial colorings

    ◊ Monosodium glutamate (MSG)

    ◊ Table salt

◆ **Eat consistently.**

When you ignore your instinctual signals of hunger, many of the physical systems of the body are challenged, such as your blood sugar levels. There is a natural rhythm to eating which supports your health and energy. By regularly eating throughout the day and fasting in the evening and at night, you will be encouraging optimum health and well-being.

◆ **Pay attention to quality vs. quantity.**

When it comes to food, the quality is of much greater significance than the quantity. What tends to happen when the food quality is poor is that the body is left searching for vital nutrients and this can trigger a response to eat more. By choosing high quality ingredients, the body will be nourished and your appetite and cravings will be balanced.

◆ **Question your food cravings.**

◊ In some situations, craving a certain food is a signal that the body needs a specific nutrient. When pregnant women crave ice cream and pickles, their body or the baby is craving calcium, which comes from the ice cream, and the vinegar in the pickles helps leach calcium from the mother's bones for the baby. There are healthier ways to absorb calcium, such as leafy greens!

◊ Instead of just indulging the craving, pause to figure out what your body might need, and give it the healthiest choice you can. It may even be calling for rest or water rather than food.

◊ Often, when women are craving sugar or caffeine, it is because of exhaustion. In this situation, a piece of protein would actually be a better choice.

◊ Craving chocolate during your period is a sign that you need magnesium; therefore, a supplement might be in order.

◆ **Make loving choices.**

As you navigate through this journey of making changes to how and possibly, what you are eating, choose to do it out of love for yourself. Whenever you nourish your body, you are performing a loving act. Each time you eat vegetables, you are giving yourself the nutrients that you need and this can be seen as a nurturing act of love.

HOW TO EAT
Rest and digest.

*O*bviously what you eat is of vital importance, such as which types of oils or salts you use and how you prepare vegetables. Yet one of the most significant aspects of healthy eating is actually, whether the body has the ability to assimilate and digest the food. This relates directly to the state of the nervous system, not just the health of your digestive system.

The human body has two branches to its autonomic nervous system. The first is the sympathetic, which is often called 'fight or flight' and deals with stress.

This part of the nervous system is triggered when your survival is at risk. The breath becomes shallow and the blood pumps away from the digestive tract preparing the body to either defend itself or run. When the body is in this state, the digestive system is not available to do its job. All the body's energy is going elsewhere. This survival instinct is often ignited by situations such as being late, unprepared, overwhelmed, tired, nervous, and angry or at odds with someone or something. It does not have to be a life-threatening situation; it just needs to be perceived as one. This state is more common than most people think.

When you eat in this state, the food is not properly digested and therefore the nutrients are not assimilated. It is classic to have a nervous stomach when under pressure. This is the direct result of stress on the digestive system.

In contrast, the second branch of the autonomic nervous system is the parasympathetic or the 'rest and digest' as it is also known. As it describes, the body is resting, the breath is slower, the digestive system is turned on and the whole body is prepared to digest and assimilate food and receive all the nutrients being offered. When the body is in this state, it is receptive, calm, restful and balanced: the perfect state in which to consume and digest food. The following is a list of ways to bring the body back to its 'rest and digest' state, therefore preparing it to absorb all the nutrients from food. This is especially important if you have been on the run for a few hours, triggering your 'fight or flight' response.

How To Rest And Digest:

◆ **Sit down to eat.**

This naturally stops the body motion, promotes rest and the ability to digest.

◆ **Take a few deep breaths.**

This automatically softens the belly and helps the body to drop back into 'rest and digest' mode.

◆ **Choose a calm eating environment.**

This includes not having stressful conversations while eating either in person or on the phone and not watching scary or overly emotional television shows or movies while trying to digest food. The body will naturally hold its breath at these times, disabling the digestive system.

◆ **Focus on eating.**

Be conscious not to multitask while you eat. This includes driving, walking, reading, answering the phone, using electronic gadgets or computers.

◆ **Say Grace.**

For some people reciting a simple prayer of gratitude or saying Grace before eating will naturally and effortlessly invoke a state of calm serenity, perfect for digestion.

CHEWING

slow it down.

You may remember at least once in your life someone telling you to slow down and chew your food. Well, it was not just to annoy you. Your teeth are the body's first tool in breaking food down into a substance, which can be readily absorbed by your cells. This process is a vital component of healthy digestion as the main reason to eat is to nourish your body.

The more you chew, the more the food disintegrates, which increases its surface area allowing the enzymes in the mouth and stomach to start working more efficiently. Think of the stomach as a washing machine. It churns the food up, but has no teeth.

If there is a chunk of food in there, the enzymes and churning can only break it down so much, and then the rest of the digestive system has to deal with a food particle that is too big. By chewing a meal well, especially proteins, the rest of the digestive system does not have to work so hard; therefore, there is less chance of particles becoming stuck and putrefied. This also reduces the risk of constipation.

The question is how much chewing is enough?

This really depends on what you are eating. A banana certainly does not need as much chewing as a piece of meat, yet all foods should be broken down into tiny particles. This usually entails about twenty to thirty chews. The idea is for the food to be in liquid-form before it is swallowed.

Chewing well also helps in making you more aware of what you are actually eating and what you are ingesting. Another benefit is that it brings more consciousness to the environment and discourages the multitasking habits, which often collaborate with inhaling your food!

"I always find when I sit down to eat and consciously chew, I tend to have fewer food cravings later on. Also when I am out to eat with friends I am always a little envious of really slow eaters because they are still enjoying their food when my plate is empty!" ~ Miranda

EATING REGULAR MEALS

Fueling the tank.

Breakfast Fit For A Queen Or King.

As the name suggests, breakfast is about 'breaking the fast' from the previous day. Ideally, this would mean you have not eaten since the night before or sundown. This first meal of the day is meant to switch the body back on. Assume that you wake up at about six or seven in the morning. If you do not eat until eleven or twelve, this would be considered an early lunch; therefore, you have actually missed breakfast, the most important meal of the day and may not have actually eaten for about fifteen hours.

As the old saying goes, 'eat breakfast fit for a King or Queen,' meaning this should be your biggest meal of the day: healthy, balanced and nutritious with enough sustenance to energize the body until lunchtime. This does not mean a sugar fest of coffee and doughnuts! What is being recommended is a combination of protein, fruit, yogurt, unrefined grains or even soup or vegetables.

You may find that you are not hungry first thing in the morning, because your body is used to skipping breakfast. You may even skip breakfast; eat a light to medium lunch and a feast for dinner. The problem with this scenario is that the food from dinner then sits in the digestive tract overnight and the calories are not used up for activity. Nighttime is the natural resting phase for the digestive system; therefore eating heavily later in the day can actually put a strain on the body. This pattern also stalls the liver and can leave you with a feeling of lethargy and fullness upon waking, which may lead you to skip breakfast again. This pattern of eating can also cause weight gain. Commit to eating a healthy breakfast and give your body the proper fuel and energy to feel strong and balanced throughout the day.

"I am a strong advocate for eating healthy unconventional foods for breakfast that would usually be considered appropriate for lunch or dinner. Leftovers are one of my favorites. They often taste better the next day." ~ Miranda

Lunch Fit For A Princess Or Prince.

In an ideal world, you have already eaten a hearty healthy breakfast. Within four hours or less the body will need to be refueled again and lunch is a perfect opportunity to bring in an abundance of vegetables. Depending on the amount of physical activity planned for the rest of the day, some high-quality protein is a good idea to fuel the fire for later in the day. Eating protein is especially important if you experience an energy lull between three and four in the afternoon.

Dinner Fit For A Peasant.

For many, dinner is the favorite meal, filled with rich, heavy and comforting foods. This is especially true if breakfast was missed, because the body is then desperately searching for more calories. The trouble is, these calories are not going to be used, which can result in weight gain and problems with a heavily taxed digestive system.

An ideal peasant dinnertime meal, however unappealing that may sound, might consist of soup and salad, or steamed vegetables with a small amount of protein. Keep in mind that dinner will ideally be the smallest meal of the day, therefore keep it light. This will not be so hard if you have eaten a substantial breakfast and lunch.

"There are nights that I eat a delicious, rich meal with friends and it is worth its weight in gold. But if this can be balanced with eating as nature intended, the rest of the time I receive the gift of feeling light, hungry and energized the next morning."
~ Miranda

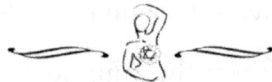

True healthcare reform starts in your kitchen, not in Washington."
~Anonymous

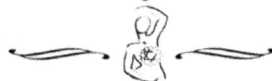

WATER

Liquid life force.

Once upon a time there was a riverbed.

The rains kept a continual flow of water running throughout her banks.

This current allowed for any build-up of residue to be gently washed away.

But, over time, the rains ceased, a drought came and the waters started to dry up.

The river ceased to flow, the animals stopped coming and debris started to build up

in the riverbed. Mosquitoes came and laid their eggs in the stagnant pools.

The remains of dead fish rotted at the edges of shallow puddles.

Flies swarmed, litter was dropped.

Yet there was nothing to help cleanse this torrid waste.

Then, after what seemed an eternity, the rains came.

A torrent starting high up in the mountains.

The riverbed welcomed the water, her mouth open wide.

As the liquid life force rushed through her walls she became cleansed and purified.

All the dust and dirt was washed away.

New life was formed and the old way was restored.

Once again there was a flow, a cleansing, a re-hydration and replenishing.

So let the rains come.

It is quite extraordinary, given how solid you might feel, that in reality so much of you is liquid. With this in mind, the water that you drink not only replenishes your cells,
but it also helps to keep the body cleansed and healthy, just like the riverbed. You can live for days, weeks even, without any food; but a couple of days without water and the body will die. When you do not drink enough, your internal organs dry out. By the time your mouth and skin are parched, the inner organs are already in trouble.

Therefore, drink water. It really is that simple! For some, this is easier said than done. If you tend not to get thirsty, hours can go by without even a drop passing your lips. If this is the case, form some kind of discipline around drinking water.

How To Increase Your Water Consumption:

◆ Set a timer to remind yourself to drink every two to three hours.

◆ Have bottles or glasses of water nearby such as on your desk, by your bed and in your car.

◆ Keep a list of how much you drink each day. It can be shocking to see how little you may actually have consumed.

◆ Fill a big water bottle and set an intention to drink it by midday.

◆ Drink two to three cups in the first few hours of waking when the body is most dehydrated.

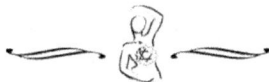

"water is the driving force in nature."
~ Leonardo Da Vinci

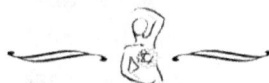

The Whys And Wherefores Of Water:

◆ Dehydration is a major cause of constipation.

◆ Water is your most effective and cheapest form of detoxifying the body.

◆ As soon as anything is added to water, the body recognizes it as food.

◆ The ultimate re-hydration, good old-fashioned, pure water is your best medicine.

◆ Choose a clean source for your water, such as a high quality filter system.

◆ Water in glass bottles is also good, but try to avoid tap water.

◆ Water should be drunk at room temperature. It is less shocking for the body.

◆ Eliminate ice cold drinks with a meal, as they slow down the digestive process.

◆ Food does not pass into the intestine until it is body temperature.

◆ In addition, cold drinks solidify fats eaten, making them harder to digest.

◆ Only consume small amounts of water with a meal; otherwise, it dilutes the digestive enzymes and the food is not broken down properly, which can cause problems further on in the digestive tract.

◆ It is more beneficial to drink smaller amounts of water more frequently since the body can only absorb a certain amount at a time. The body is extremely thirsty after a night's sleep. Therefore, drink plenty on waking. This also helps to bring the body into a more alkaline condition.

◆ A cup of warm water in the morning helps with elimination.

◆ If water is stored in plastic bottles and is subjected to heat, such as being left in a car on a hot day, the plastic molecules leech into the water, which you then consume. Avoid this by using glass bottles that are made to withstand heat.

◆ Plastic bottles of water are not designed to be used a second time.

◆ The plastic is cheap and not durable.

◆ If you buy water in plastic bottles, be sure it is stored somewhere cool and out of direct sunlight. This includes the large water bottles that are delivered to your sunny doorstep!

How Much Water Is Enough?

This is a good question. How much water should you actually be drinking? It is often said to drink eight glasses a day. However, in reality, it depends on the weather, the amount of physical activity you do and how much water you drank the day before. The best suggestion is to monitor your urine. The only time this does not work is when certain supplements, such as B vitamins are taken. They tend to turn the urine a strong yellow.

◆ Normally urine should be a pale yellow color.

◆ If it is a stronger color, you need to drink more water.

◆ Urine should not smell. If it does, it is a sign that it is too concentrated or that your body is trying to cleanse or detox. Either way, drink more water.

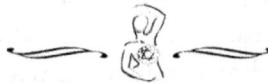

"We never know the worth of water till the well is dry."
~ Thomas Fuller

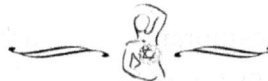

SALT

Salt of the earth and sea.

Along with water, salt is another of life's essentials and also one of the most popular and widely-used condiments. Animals and humans will cross deserts and travel miles to find salt. The origin of its name comes from the word 'salary' showing the essential worth and importance of this simple white powder, which was so precious that people were willing to be paid with it.

How many times have you thought, 'It just needs a pinch of salt.'

This compound seems to bring out the natural flavor of other ingredients, also adding a stimulation of its own. Yet, too much salt makes food unpalatable. Therefore, much of this seasoning's impact is in getting the perfectly balanced amount. Too much can make you thirsty and crave sweets; not enough can leave the body mineral-deficient, creating a lack of vitality, stagnation and the inability to think clearly.

You may have noticed that when you eat very salty foods such as potato chips, you then crave something sweet, like a soda or a piece of fruit. This is the body's way of trying to re-address its balance. Think of the body as a teeter-totter or seesaw. The salt heavily weighs down one end, and then the sugar catapults you to the other. If this happens too often, it can cause excessive stress on the body. The answer is to try not to live in extremes and to figure out what is the right amount of salt for you. One of the easiest ways is to notice if you are craving something sweet after eating salt. That is a sign that maybe what you just ate was a little on the salty side.

Even more important than the amount of salt, is the type you use.

The majority of salts offered in restaurants and markets are regular table salt. What has been done to this product is one of the biggest food crimes of all. Just like sugar and flour, salt has also been heavily refined. What is called salt nowadays has been so highly processed, bleached and modified, its effect on the body is more like that of a poison than a nutrient. In fact, all of the essential components have been removed, leaving it deficient in the minerals needed for the body to absorb the sodium that is essential for life.

Unrefined salt, on the other hand, which has been processed naturally, is abundant in many of the trace minerals that the body needs. This means it has been left to dry in the sun and mined and packaged without processing. Naturally, mined salt also has much more flavor. The good news is you need less as the taste is stronger and cleaner and it enhances the flavors already in the food.

To switch to a good quality salt is actually one of the easiest, cheapest and most life-enhancing steps you can take to improve your health.

Key Points To Look For When Choosing Salt Are:

◆ Unrefined

◆ Sundried

◆ No heat processing

◆ No additives or preservatives

◆ Unbleached

◆ Hand or naturally harvested

Beneficial salt is taken directly from the earth or sea. It is naturally processed, dried, and simply packaged to fit in a container. It therefore remains abundant in all the trace minerals the body needs. High quality salt will harmonize and stabilize the body.

The amount of salt you use depends on which type you have chosen. High quality sea salt has a much stronger flavor. Therefore, if you are following a recipe, which calls for regular table salt, and you want to substitute, cut the amount by about half. You can always add more if needed.

It is easier on the body to absorb the minerals from salt if it has been cooked, therefore it is more beneficial to add the high quality salt earlier on in the recipe instead of sprinkling at the table.

The amount of salt you use is certainly a personal taste. Feel free to add or subtract the amount you use in cooking.

Your palette is your ultimate guide.

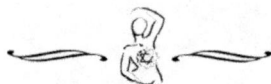

"Let yourself be open and life will be easier.
A spoon of salt in a glass of water
makes the water undrinkable.
A spoon of salt in a lake is almost unnoticed."
~ Buddha

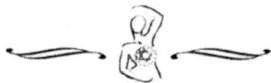

THE VERSATILE VEGETABLE
The food of the Gods.

Vegetables, with all their different colors, shapes, sizes and textures, not to mention smells and flavors, are extraordinarily versatile and display the adaptability of these extraordinary plants. These are good reasons why vegetables, along with chocolate, can be called 'The food of the Gods.' The choices are endless these days. You no longer have to be limited by seasonal changes, as most vegetables are grown all year round. This helps you add more vegetables to your daily food choices.

Reasons To Increase Your Vegetable Intake:

◆ **Nutritional value**

Vegetables are literally packed with nutrients, vitamins and minerals. There are many wonderful and informative books written on their nutritional breakdown, if that interests you. Yet, what is being recommended here is a basic increase in your daily consumption of vegetables. The way whole foods are so perfectly balanced and designed is very different to a compact little pill that is exactly the right size to swallow. In addition, yes, you could take a pill. Yet, there are vitamins and minerals which science is still discovering in vegetables and fresh foods. You are greatly increasing your chances of getting all that you need by going back to what nature intended.

◆ **Vitality and life-force**

The life force, energy and vitality of vegetables by far surpasses that of any processed food. Whenever you buy vegetables, ideally, you want to eat them within a few days or they will wilt and lose their nutritional value and also become unappetizing. The vitality of the vegetable decreases each day after it has been harvested. When you eat a fresh vegetable, you are also receiving life force. This vitality is extremely important to help feed your own essence.

◆ **Increase fiber**

Eating fiber is not all about bran, flax seed and prunes, honestly! Eating vegetables can play a major part in your daily fiber intake. Fiber is often lacking in a western diet of white flour and refined sugars. Each time you eat a vegetable, not only are you consuming quantities of fuel and nutrition for your body, you are aiding the body's basic ability to eliminate and sweep out all that is not beneficial for you. It is rather like adding peanut butter to your hair when you get chewing gum stuck in it: the whole mess washes out instantaneously. By adding a neutralizer, the problem is dissolved. Strange analogies perhaps, but without the bulk from the vegetables to help clean out toxins and residue, the body is much more prone to store and hold onto these poisons.

◆ **Balancing alkalinity**

Vegetables are alkaline-forming when consumed and digested. The reason this is important is that the body needs to be in an alkaline condition for optimal health. Therefore the more alkaline-forming foods you eat, such as fruits and vegetables, the easier it is for your system to stay healthy. Eating vegetables is a quick and easy way to achieve this. It is all about balance. The body does need some acidity and plenty is received from sources such as animal protein, sugars and grains. For good health, the percentage of alkaline-forming foods needs to be much greater than acid-forming ones.

◆ **The waist-line and money**

The good news is you will not become fat or poor eating vegetables. Pound for pound, they are much cheaper than most other foods. By filling up on a variety of vegetables and using animal products and grains as a side dish, you will not become as hungry and will be less likely to crave that cookie or piece of cake. In many dietary guidelines, vegetables do not even have a caloric value, especially the leafy green ones, so eat up and enjoy!

◈ The icing on the cake

What is being suggested here is that at least half of each meal should be made up of vegetables. For many, this may be a major shift in how you were raised and taught to eat. Many fast food restaurants may not agree, yet with all of the reasons in favor of vegetables, it is very much in your best interest to start increasing your consumption, even if it is just by a small amount each day. Vegetables tend to get a bad rap because they are not given the chance to go beyond the boiled-carrot syndrome. Yet, given some imagination and a book full of flavorful recipes, a carrot can be caramelized, pureed, baked or sautéed and utterly transformed into a delicious part of any meal.

◈ A step by step transition

Now for the nitty-gritty. How does one leap from a salad every other day to eating vegetables at each meal? The answer is baby steps. Each day add one more portion of vegetables. If you are not used to eating so many, start by adding soup or other cooked varieties. This will help with digestion and assimilation. Vary how you prepare your vegetables. Eat some raw salads in the middle of the day, especially in the summer. Take the time to roast, steam or sauté your vegetables. The more variation you have, the better. Rotating types of vegetables is important too. Do not be stuck in a rut of sautéing spinach night after night, otherwise, you will get tired of it and never want to eat spinach again. The transition to the more starchy vegetables, such as potatoes, corn, carrots and all kinds of squashes, is usually easier, but remember to include many leafy greens along the way. Adding food enzymes can also be beneficial.

THE PROTOCOL OF PROTEIN
why eat protein?

Protein provides what the body utilizes for energy and to repair itself. It is vital for developing and maintaining muscle mass and is essential for making hormones, antibodies, enzymes and tissue. It also helps the body to maintain a healthy balance between acid and alkaline. Yet, like anything in life, too much can be harmful, as it makes the body overly acidic and can stress the kidneys and urinary tract.

As you can see, it is all about balance and listening to the intelligence of your body.

A good illustration, which highlights protein's effectiveness at giving you energy, is to imagine you are building a fire. The kindling and newspaper are the refined and simple carbohydrates, such as white sugar and flour. They give you a surge of energy as they burst into flames, yet do not last. Fruits, vegetables, and whole-grains are like small dry logs. They catch fire easily and burn for a little while. When it comes to eating proteins or fats, it is as though you are placing a big, heavy log on the fire. In the right environment, protein will burn and give off heat for a good few hours, sustaining and giving you and your body the gift of energy.

The other benefit of protein is that it can reduce sugar cravings. The next time you are longing for something sweet, try eating a small piece of protein instead. It will actually give you more energy, balance your blood sugar levels and stop the sugar craving cycle. As you may have noticed, eating sugar tends to trigger the yearning for even more sugar.

When it comes to eating animal proteins, the most important factor is to make sure the nutrients can be absorbed and the waste products eliminated. There are a number of ways to optimize the body's ability to digest protein and therefore increase your capacity to receive what is needed for energy and repair.

The Protocol Of Digesting Protein:

◆ **Chew the protein thoroughly.**

Chewing your food well enables the first stage of digestion to work properly, which is in your mouth. This action breaks down the protein into small particles, thus making a greater surface area for the enzymes in your saliva to work. This relieves the amount of work to be done by the other systems in the body.

◆ **Combine protein with plenty of vegetables.**

Animal protein is acid forming. Therefore, adding vegetables helps keep a more alkaline environment in the body, which is essential for health and well-being.

◆ **Choose organic and pasture-fed animal products.**

By choosing high quality protein, the body does not have to work so hard to eliminate all the toxins and pesticides. Also, if animals are allowed to roam freely on green pastures, the meat will be higher in beneficial nutrients, which are absent in grain-fed animals.

◆ **Eat protein as a condiment.**

To receive the greatest benefits from eating proteins use it as a complement to the main dish. This in an ideal world would consist mainly of vegetables. Although protein is vital to the body in certain amounts, too much can cause an acidic condition and is hard to digest. When eating protein with your meal, keep the quantity to about a quarter of the plate or the size of the palm of your hand.

◆ **Vary the types of protein.**

Each type of protein has different qualities; therefore, it is best to rotate proteins, such as fish, meat or eggs enabling your body to get a wider range of nutrients. This allows the body to send you a message if it is reacting unfavorably to a certain kind.

◆ **Cook protein slowly on a low heat.**

Another option is to cook protein slowly, in casseroles, slow-cookers or croc pots. This makes the protein easier to break down and assimilate.

◆ **Prepare protein as raw or rare as possible.**

Once protein is cooked, it is harder to digest. In addition, many of the enzymes needed to break it down are destroyed by heat. It is essential to cook certain proteins such as chicken but, fish or eggs are more beneficial eaten lightly cooked or raw.

◆ **Eat protein with cultured foods.**

In many cultures, eating fermented foods is a normal part of the meal, such as Kimchee in Korean cuisine or Miso soup in Japanese. When cultured or fermented foods are eaten with protein, they aid digestion by adding a surplus of enzymes and friendly bacteria. This helps the protein molecules to be broken down more efficiently.

◆ **Take digestive enzymes with the meal.**

Digestive enzymes are particularly helpful if out with friends or at a restaurant where the food choices are challenging. This helps the body by making sure there are plenty of enzymes available, especially if combining protein with a starch.

◆ Eat heavier protein between 11 am and 2 pm.

This is the most beneficial time for the body to digest protein. If you eat a heavy protein later in the day, it can negatively affect your sleep and your body's ability to digest efficiently.

◆ Combine protein with non-starchy foods and vegetables.

This is about which foods complement each other when eaten together and which foods are better eaten separately. To put it very simply, the body uses certain enzymes to digest concentrated protein, such as a piece of chicken and a different group of enzymes to digest concentrated starches, such as a potato. Many foods have a combination of proteins and carbohydrates in them, but it is the concentrated forms, which are best eaten separately. Therefore, when you sit down to a meal of chicken and potatoes, these different enzymes are mixed together. Unfortunately, each group of enzymes has a different effect. The protein enzymes form an acidic environment, while the starch enzymes form an alkaline one. They neutralize each other, leaving the body with a lack of working enzymes to break down your meal. If you are having a problem with your digestion, the simple act of combining your foods appropriately is one of the easiest ways to reduce reactions from foods.

THE COMPLEX CARB

Just as a complicated woman can be a good thing, so it is with a complex carb.

It may never have occurred to you that carbohydrates are rather like women; complex, complicated yet absolutely delectably delicious. Confused as to what is a good carb and what is a bad one? Take heart, it is about to be explained.

Simple carbohydrates are also known as simple sugars and are often refined. Yet they also include fruit and milk sugars. Out of the choices fruit is the richest and most beneficial source, however, simple carbohydrates are the ones to limit or avoid.

In comparison, a complex carbohydrate forms a longer molecular string of sugars and is broken down in the body at a slower rate, giving you fuel for an extended period of time. Complex carbohydrates include sugars from vegetables, whole grains, peas and beans and they retain their nutritional value. The bottom line is increase the complex carbs and limit the simple ones.

Carbohydrates are a vital food group as they are one of the main sources of fuel for the body's cells and brain. Therefore when choosing carbohydrates it is vital to select unrefined ones, such as fruits, vegetables, beans and whole grains, as opposed to processed carbohydrates, such as sweetened drinks, desserts, candy, white flour, white rice and sugar.

An additional benefit of eating unrefined carbohydrates is that they contain fiber. Fiber is vital for reducing constipation and in turn aids in detoxifying the body.

Just as you are discovering how to love yourself, as complex as you may be, so it is with a complex carbohydrate.

CLEANSING
spring-cleaning the body.

Cleansing is one of the body's most natural and powerful methods of keeping healthy. As toxins build, there are many different systems to help flush them out and eliminate them. The problem occurs when the influx of toxins is too heavy and the possible channels of cleansing are either over-loaded or unavailable.

Imagine you have a closet that is packed full of stuff. You remember the last time you opened the door; you slammed it shut and heaved a sigh of relief that the door remained closed. Well, if you never open that door again, the junk remains, slowly accumulating more dust and possibly acquiring a few parasites. Rats, spiders and moths seem to love undisturbed mess! Yet if one day you choose to open the door, then the opportunity arises for cleaning. The body is no different.

The physical form needs to be given the same opportunity; it needs the time and tools to work through its highly intelligent process of cleansing. This could be through sweating or a bowel movement. Even illness can be a way for the body to eliminate unwanted material. Producing mucus or throwing up is a natural way of getting rid of harmful bacteria and potential poison.

Ways To Cleanse The Body:

◆ **Drink a glass of hot water and fresh lemon juice upon waking.**

This will cleanse the liver. Brush your teeth afterwards to protect tooth enamel.

◆ **Drink or eat 1 tablespoon of ground flax seed daily.**

Always combine with 8 ounces of pure water to help cleanse the colon.

◆ **Increase your intake of fresh fruits and vegetables.**

Reduce the amount of protein, refined and processed products for three full days. This will alkalize the body, helping it to detoxify.

◆ **Stop eating by 7 pm in the evening.**

This allows the body to fast until morning, which gives the digestive system and other organs time to rest.

◆ **Increase your daily intake of water.**

Drink 8 to 12 glasses of pure water a day. This will rehydrate the body and encourage the cells to eliminate toxins.

◆ **If prone to Urinary Tract Infections drink a cocktail of:**

2 ounces. of unsweetened cranberry juice, 1 teaspoon unfiltered apple cider vinegar and 1 tablespoon of lemon juice with 8 ounces of pure water in the morning. This will cleanse the kidneys and urinary tract.

◆ **Drink 2 to 3 cups of Beiller's Broth a day.**

This is a simple way to cleanse the liver and increase your daily intake of vegetables. You can find this recipe by searching "Beiler's Broth" online.

◆ **Fast for twenty-four hours.**

Only ingest liquids such as water, fruit and vegetable juices, vegetable soups and broths. Choose a day when your workload is minimal and you can rest.

◆ **Take a hot bath.**

Use one pound of Epsom salts and one pound of baking soda and soak for twenty minutes. This clears toxins out of the body. Drink 8 ounces of water afterwards.

◆ **Give yourself a full day of rest.**

Take a day and night and do nothing. Sleep, lounge around, nap, whatever it takes to achieve a deep and restful relaxation in which you achieve nothing! This gives the body time to heal.

◆ **Exercise until you sweat.**

Move the body on a regular basis to the point of sweating and being out of breath. This only needs to be done twelve minutes a day for optimum results.

◆ **Always cleanse the colon first.**

Only cleanse other organs once the colon is eliminating efficiently.

Purifying the body is a vital part of overall health.

HEALTHY CONVENIENCE FOODS

choosing to eat real food daily.

*E*very one has moments when time is of the essence. Yet this does not mean that you have to compromise your health. Whenever possible, incorporate a living fruit or vegetable into the mix. It is always a good idea to have healthy snack foods and water readily available. Hunger and low blood sugar can make you cranky and impedes your ability to discern good foods from bad. Remember too, that sometimes the body may be thirsty and not hungry.

Some Simple And Accessible Ideas For Food On The Go:

◆ Fresh or dried fruits

◆ Fresh, raw vegetables

◆ Trail mix, nuts or seeds

◆ Healthy bars

◆ Nut butters with fruit or vegetables

◆ Hummus and raw vegetables

◆ Guacamole or salsa with corn chips

◆ Apple and goat or sheep cheese

◆ Live yogurt, Bio K or kefir

◆ Live yogurt or kefir with fresh fruit and flax seed

◆ Smoothies with fresh fruit and kefir

◆ Ready washed greens and salads

◆ Cultured vegetables

◆ Olives

◆ Edaname

- Soups
- Vegetable chips
- Seaweed snacks
- Kale crisps
- Boiled eggs
- Smoked salmon and goat cheese
- Sliced meats
- Healthy left-overs

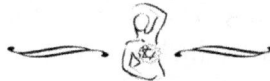

"Healthy is merely the slowest rate at which one can die!"
~ Anonymous

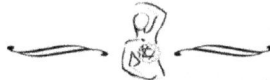

SIMPLICITY FOR COMPLICATED TIMES

The versatile vegetable is more than just a cookbook,
it is a comprehensive guide for nourishing your life.

For more detailed nutritional information, guidance and delicious yet simple recipes, please enjoy reading the vital and life enhancing information in Miranda's book 'The Food of Life, The Versatile Vegetable.' Incorporate the recipes to spice up and increase your vegetable intake. Practice implementing what you have read throughout the rest of your life.

For example, while reading about 'chewing', the goal is to chew every mouthful thirty times and become aware of how this affects your energy levels, your digestion, elimination, and appetite. If you tend to inhale your food, this will seem slow, frustrating, and possibly annoying. Hang in there and know this new habit will encourage you to sit down to eat, which is one of the other topics and to eat less. This is always good for the waistline and inner thighs! Keep practicing this new habit and slowly incorporate other new choices into your life when you are ready. Some will be much more challenging than others will.

Just notice.

Do not judge.

This is your life in process.

The beauty is during this experience of exploring food, your body will become healthier and you will become intimately aware of the benefits of eating nourishing food. As you **willingly** consume these healthier choices, you can release having to avoid that which is not good for you.

This transition from willfulness to willingness can change your life.

"Miranda works on the ancient Hippocratic principle "Let food be thy medicine and medicine be thy food" - namely, we can bring tremendous health benefits and vastly reduce disease if we make the best possible decisions around what we choose to nourish our body. The Versatile Vegetable is a gentle and well-organized introduction for both experienced vegetarians and hearty carnivores who are flirting with the idea of introducing more vegetables into their diet. The book helpfully introduces all of the basic cooking concepts, and has lots of easy-to-prepare ideas; she proves that a healthy diet need not be costly nor complicated, but it is our natural right to feel healthy, nourished and happy...and food is a crucial contributing factor!" ~ Marcus Freed

To order 'The Food of Life, The Versatile Vegetable',
please visit Miranda's web site at
www.MirandaJBarrett.com /resources/the-food-of-life-books.

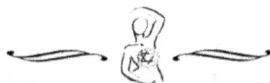

"In a world of growing consciousness
around the medical benefits of good food choices,
The versatile vegetable is a welcome addition to the recipe bookshelf."

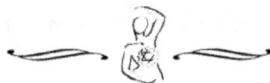

REVEAL MORE TRUTH

If it is good for you, the chances are you will feel nourished.

This precious time is about exploring your relationship with food. This can be a loaded and highly emotional subject, particularly if you tend to choose ice cream or chocolate as your comforter, over a slightly less cuddly plate of vegetables!

As you explore the world of 'Nourishing Nutrition', remember that you are gathering information. This allows you to inquire deeper into the self and get a clear picture of the patterns that are working and the habits that are not. Be kind, non-judgmental and loving with yourself. Some of these habits may have been instilled in you years ago. Rather than rip them out in a bloody mess, I encourage you to replace them lovingly with a new thought and a more nourishing choice.

LOVING SUPPORT FOR YOUR SELF-CARE:

◆ Fill in the Daily Food Chart.

Go to *www.MirandaJBarrett.com/resources/nourishing-nutrition* to print out additional copies of the food chart. It is fascinating that as soon as you start to reintroduce foods from the avoid list, you will no longer want to write your confessions down! Pay attention to this and write it anyway. It is when you become conscious and accountable that change can occur.

◆ Follow 'The Daily Practice' as a way to incorporate the teachings.

◆ Keep your kitchen stocked with healthy, live and nutritious foods.

If there is no chocolate to be found, then it is harder to eat. Do not shop when you are hungry. Your cravings will be bigger than your calorie burning abilities.

◆ **Be mindful about getting enough sleep, rest and moving the body.**

Remember these are the other two vital components of 'The Foundational Trinity.' Keep all three within your awareness.

Nourishing yourself can be received in many different ways. What I am offering here is for you to pause at any given moment to notice what would truly restore and nurture you. This could range from a nap to a piece of fruit or a glass of water.

Your body thanks you in advance, as do I, for giving yourself the gift of nourishing your body as a temple and a sacred place, which houses your being. In any moment, you can step towards or away from health. Every time you choose a nurturing act towards yourself, I encourage you to celebrate and acknowledge this accomplishment.

I look forward to connecting with you as we conclude 'The Foundational Trinity' of sleep, nutrition and movement in the next book, **'Embodying Movement'** which will allow you to restore balance in your life and discover how to embrace your whole being through the life enhancing benefits of body movement.

Sending love to you on this journey of truly nourishing yourself,

Miranda

It is what you eat, not what you avoid,
that nourishes and heals your body.

CHARTS, CHARTS, GLORIOUS CHARTS

"Let food be thy medicine and medicine be thy food"
~ Hippocrates

This Honest Daily Food Study will bring a whole new level of awareness and consciousness to the foundation of your life. In addition, will give you clarity beyond measure on what is working in your world and what is not.

◆ Please go to **www.MirandaJBarrett.com /resources/nourishing-nutrition** to print out more copies for yourself. Give yourself the gift of seeing your relationship to food clearly laid out in front of you.

◆ Fill out the **Honest Daily Food Study** on a daily basis until you begin to see your patterns and your own relationship with food.

◆ Ask yourself the powerful question: Are my food habits giving me more energy or is what I am putting in my body, weighing me down?

◆ Once you are clear about your basic food needs and see the importance of honoring this vital aspect of your life, lovingly make the necessary adjustments to replenish and nurture yourself.

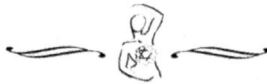

*"He who distinguishes the true savor of his food
can never be a glutton; he who does not cannot be otherwise."*
~ Thoreau

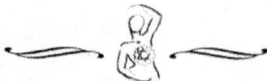

AN HONEST DAILY FOOD STUDY

Day: Date:

	BREAKFAST	LUNCH	DINNER	SNACKS
What did you eat for:				
Were you hungry?				
Did you sit down to eat?				
Did you multi-task?				
Did you chew well?				
How did you feel afterwards?				
How many servings of vegetables?				
How many servings of protein?				
How much water did you drink?				
How much caffeine did you drink?				
How much alcohol did you drink?				
How many sodas did you drink?				
Did you finish eating by 7:00 pm?				
Did you take any supplements?				
How do you feel about your relationship with food today?				
… and love yourself anyway.				

Give yourself the gift of seeing your food relationship clearly laid out in front of you.

Please go to
www.MirandaJBarrett.com /resources/nourishing-nutrition
to print out more copies for yourself.

ABOUT MIRANDA

A spirited guide and mentor.

Miranda is a passionate and devoted leader. Her loving and wise support will guide you on a transformational journey as her powerful teachings unveil the truth of who you are. Her gift is to offer potent tools, which inspire exquisite and beautiful self-care and empower you to live the fullest and most authentic life possible. As a mentor and guide, Miranda deeply walks her talk and is fearless about her own path of self-discovery, as she weaves the sacred into the mundane.

The simple, yet powerful premise offered by the mystic Rumi is the foundation of Miranda's philosophy and mission:

"Never give from the depths of your well,
always give from your overflow."

Miranda gives Council and Guidance for the Mind, Body and Spirit. With a background in Nutrition and Energy work, Miranda is the Creator of 'A Woman's Truth' and 'The Spirit of Energy', an Author, a Workshop and Retreat Leader, a Reiki Master and Yoga and Meditation teacher. Miranda studies under the guidance of her Beloved teachers Rod Stryker and Adyashanti.

To speak with or follow Miranda, please call or visit:

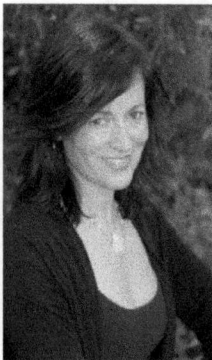

Phone: 626~798~6544
eMail: Info@MirandaJBarrett.com
Website: www.MirandaJBarrett.com
Facebook: Miranda J Barrett
Twitter: MirandaJBarrett

ABOUT HELENA

A visionary artist.

Helena Nelson-Reed is a visionary artist whose primary medium is watercolor. Born in Seattle, Washington, she was raised in Marin County and Napa Valley, California and today lives in Illinois. A largely self-taught artist whose educational emphasis and degree is in psychology, Nelson-Reed's primary focus is exploring the collective consciousness and the portrayal of archetypal imagery in the tradition of Carl Jung and Joseph Campbell. Rendered in luminous watercolor technique often described as ephemeral, Nelson-Reed's paintings are created in extraordinary detail, pushing the medium of watercolor past the usual limits. Her work may be found in private collections, book covers, magazines and CD covers. Nelson-Reed also has a line of jewelry, calendars and greeting cards.

Helena's Mission:

My images can be interpreted many ways, and for some will serve as portal to the mythic landscape. Descriptions providing background about each painting are available by request. Navigating and translating myth into contemporary wisdom is the traditional way of transmitting information, a shamanic and multi-cultural practice.

Myth, fairy, folk and spiritual lore describe divine beings and supernatural life forms arriving unbidden and disguised. In our earthly dimension, mortals often play similar roles in the lives of one another. Destinies and energies collide and interact, visible and invisible forces are at work. The mythic realms are timeless, offering insight and inspiration. While my paintings have a positive energy, many have roots in the shadows of life experience and human psyche; like the lotus blossom rooted in pond mud. For many, life is one challenge followed by the next, like beads on an endless string.

Take heart! Like goddess Inanna, one may navigate the underworld, move through dark places yet return to the realms of light battle scarred but wiser, richer for the experience. Read the ancient tales, the great mythic literature; draw strength, for they are repositories of wisdom.

Visit Helena's website for her art purchase information and art to wear jewelry:

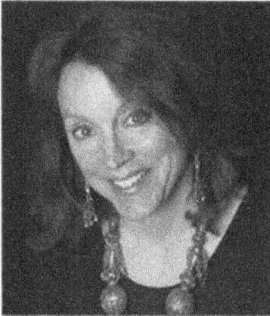

eMail: HNelsonReed@Gmail.com
Websites: www.HelenaNelsonReed.com
www.etsy.com/shop/HelenaNelsonReed
Blog: www.dancingdovestudio.blogspot.com
Facebook: MorningDove Design By Helena

MIRANDA'S WORLD

*Ways to stay connected
and aligned with your truth.*

BOOKS:

A Woman's Truth

A life truly worth living.

Priceless teachings reveal your transformational
journey ahead. Obstacles to self-care are explored
as clear and loving intentions are conceived.

The Grandeur of Sleep

Permission to rest.

Miraculous benefits are realized as the worlds of sleep,
relaxation and rejuvenation are explored and deeply honored.

Nourishing Nutrition

Reclaim your health and vitality.

Reap the bountiful rewards while eating as nature intended.
Claim your health and vitality with these simple,
yet powerful tools to nourish and heal your body.

Embodying Movement
Ground your whole being.

Restore balance in your life. Discover how to embrace
your whole being through the life-enhancing benefits of body movement.

Body Care
Cherish your body as a temple.

Learn to honor your extraordinary body
as a living temple and listen to the healing messages she whispers.

Feminine Power
Fully access your supreme birthright.

Welcome and reclaim this intrinsic privilege while living
in harmonious balance between the masculine and the feminine.

The Abundance of Wealth
Receive the gifts of prosperity.

Understand the energy flow of prosperity and weave
the threads of abundance throughout the tapestry of your life.

Find Your Authentic Voice
The courage to express who you truly are.

Your greatest ally is born
when you courageously speak your truth and claim your unique power.

Loving Yourself
A love affair with the self.

As you become highly attuned to your own needs,
allow love to lead the way. Grant yourself permission
to honor and express your heart's truest desires.
Love yourself, no matter what.

Living A Spiritual Life
Ground your divine essence here on earth.

Discover what spirituality means to you, by consciously
living between the two worlds of the sacred and the mundane.

Service As A Way Of Life
Ignite the fire of love to truly be of service.

By utilizing the gems of exquisite self-care
on a daily basis and honoring your truth, your mission of service is born.

The Crowning Glory
Fully Rejoice in Being You.

A celebration overflowing with love,
blessings, grace and gratitude. Stand confident within
your truth as your mind begins to serve your heart.

The Food Of Life
The versatile vegetable.

More than just a cookbook,
a comprehensive guide for nourishing your life.

Reiki
The spirit of Energy.

An insightful guidebook full of wisdom
which introduces you to the potent and healing world of Reiki.

CARDS:

Inspiration Cards
A daily Spiritual Practice.

Sixty-Five cards with simple yet inspirational qualities
to live by and an insightful guidebook to lead the way.

CD'S:

The Grandeur of sleep and Rejuvenating Rest

An ancient healing art of rest and relaxation.

Simple yet profound practices that alleviate stress and tension allowing your mind, body and spirit to heal, restore and replenish.

TO ORDER PLEASE VISIT:

www.MirandaJBarrett.com
www.Amazon.com

*All books are available in printed or eBook form.

TESTIMONIES

to Miranda's book 'The Food Of Life, The Versatile Vegetable'.

"The deepest, most curative effect one can make towards their health and well-being is to change how and what you are eating. 'We are what we eat' is highlighted again and again. Miranda gives us wide choices and makes healthy cooking possible in this fast-paced world."

Eileen ~ Chiropractor ~ Altadena, CA

"If you are one of the many who are now making better choices about your body, your diet, and the way you live your life, this book is timely. Following the author's wise and gently instruction will surely help you reach your goals."

Judith ~ Intuitive Healer ~ Pasadena, CA

"I was delivered to Miranda two years ago in the throes of a major health struggle. I had followed several diets, worked with many healers, and consulted with different nutritionists, but it was not until I worked with Miranda that I began to heal. Miranda is grounded, practical, and compassionate perspective on nutrition and wellness made the healing process as swift and easy as possible. I am amazed at the amount of energy I have today. It would not be possible without Miranda's loving guidance and wisdom. I am deeply grateful to her."

Kristina ~ Reiki Master ~ Santa Barbara, CA

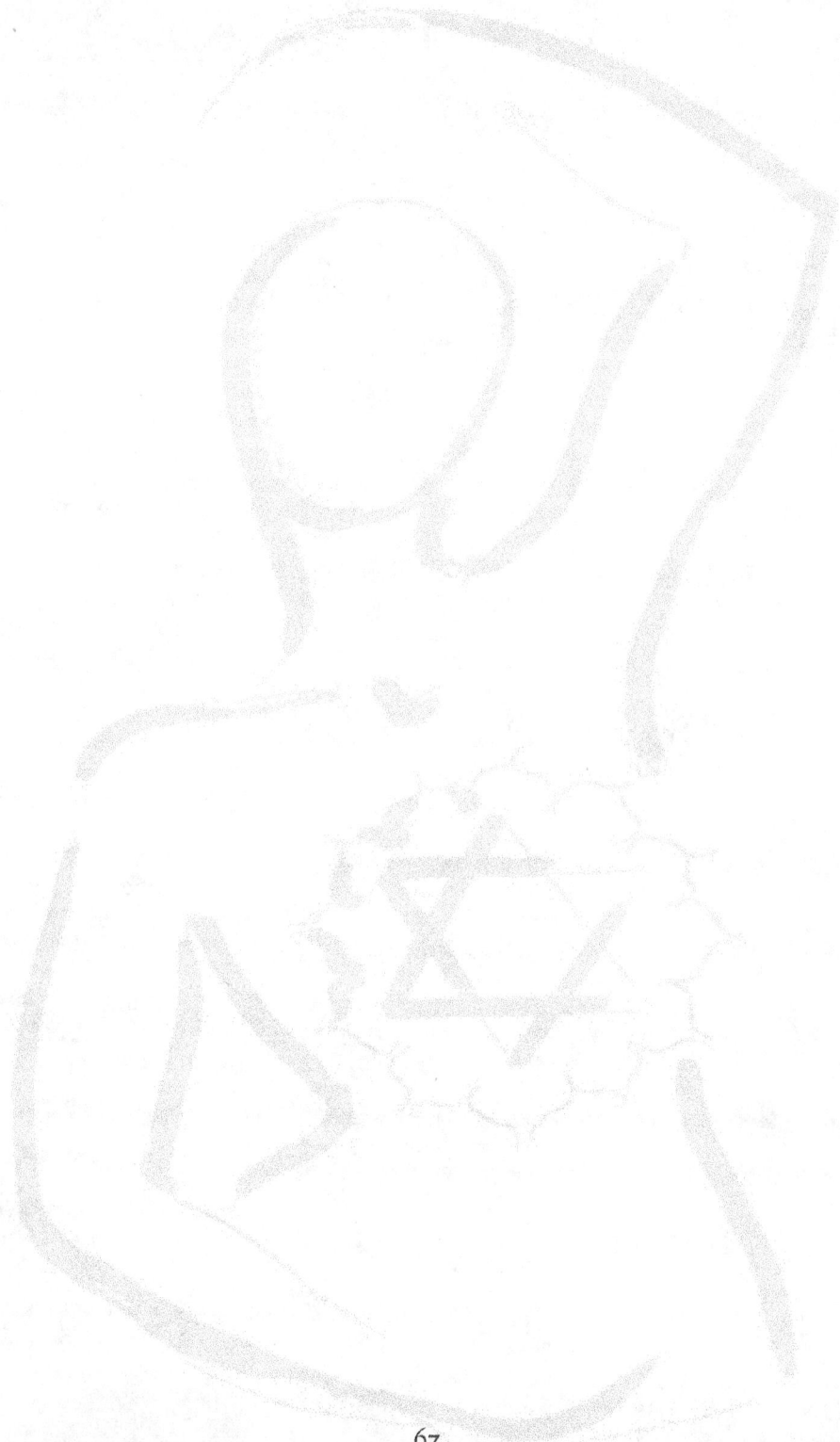

www.ingramcontent.com/pod-product-compliance
Lightning Source LLC
Chambersburg PA
CBHW081200270326

41930CB00014B/3234